Table of Contents

ALS Muscle Twitching: Characteristics and Management

1. Introduction

The physiology of muscle stiffness and muscle cramps in ALS/MND is not widely investigated as compared to muscle atrophy, muscle weakness, and muscle fasciculation. Although these symptoms are very common, very little is known about their characteristics and management. Increased knowledge and data about muscle twitching in ALS/MND would likely be valuable to the patient community. Both muscle stiffness (spasticity) and muscle cramps are the result of abnormal afferent inputs, are not due to muscle abnormality directly, and therefore should be addressed separately. In contrast, muscle twitching in ALS/MND may arise due to a combination of abnormal excitability and disinhibition in the CNS or NMJ/muscle.

Amyotrophic lateral sclerosis, or Lou Gehrig's disease, is a neurodegenerative disease that affects the motor neurons, causing muscles to weaken and atrophy. Besides muscle weakness, pain, cramping, and muscle twitching are the most common symptoms reported by ALS/MND patients. Muscle twitching can rarely be the first clinical presentation of ALS/MND, with only a few reports of patients being diagnosed solely based on muscle twitching and no other signs of motor neuron disease.

2. Understanding ALS Muscle Twitching

This simply does not happen unless the cell membrane has been mechanically or artificially disrupted. There is some evidence that a tiny disruption in one muscle cell could affect others locally, but this would not account for the typical distribution seen in motor neuron disease. The answer to why twitching happens also shows us what is key to the pathology causing death of the ALS motor neuron. As muscle fibers transmit electrical activity from cell to cell, these cell-to-cell electrical signals are amplified to "propagate." Normally, an individual muscle cell, in isolation, will not generate enough electrical energy to affect the contraction of a group of other muscle cells, even if they are really close to each other. It is clear to see that high electrical energy excitation could better drive this cell-to-cell electrical interaction, creating many such amplifications to initiate action to twitch the muscle.

Muscle twitching is an interesting phenomenon in the spectrum of muscle diseases. In the context of ALS, the twitching becomes a sufficiently important clinical hallmark that it is instrumental in diagnosis. Muscle twitching is essentially contractions but differs from the normal contractions of skeletal muscle in frequency and origin. When a skeletal muscle contracts in a way that partially ripples over the rest of the muscle, it looks like a quick flicker on the skin above it. Skeletal muscle contractions are brought forth by the release of compressed energy, as ATP is released in the last step of muscle contraction, which transiently attaches and then detaches the myosin head, so it can reach up and work again. Twitches differ in that they are actually concomitant binding of the myosin head that can translate across the whole muscle, between cells.

2.1. Definition and Causes

It is apparent that not all ALS patients develop muscle twitching at the beginning of the disease. Male patients seem to do so slightly more often than female patients. Several triggering or risk factors for muscle twitching have been suggested in the past, including exercise-related stress, caffeine intake, and smoking. In terms of ALS, muscle twitches are a very early sign, typically reported by patients up to one and up to two years before ALS is generally diagnosed, and in some cases even earlier. In rare cases, muscle twitching is observed for a very long time, sometimes up to 11 years, before other (motor) symptoms become evident, in which case the diagnosis is usually that of benign fasciculations.

Biologically, a few typical ALS mechanisms are known to be involved in muscle twitching. Specifically, protein inclusions are being formed in the muscle tissue of ALS patients, collectively related to the occurrence of muscle twitching. The formation of damaging protein oxidants of damaged mitochondria in the tissue of ALS patients has also been established. Such molecular and cellular mechanisms have not yet been related to the clinical occurrence of muscle twitches.

ALS is caused by the degeneration and death of motor neurons, some of which extend from the brain to the muscles (upper motor neurons [UMN]), and others which are responsible for muscle control within the spinal cord (lower motor neurons [LMN]). Although UMN and LMN are both affected in ALS, signs of LMN degeneration can be found in virtually all patients and are most prominent in research on deceased ALS patients. Therefore, muscle twitching is considered to result from affected lower motor neurons.

Muscle twitching is a common symptom of motor neuron diseases, the disease group within which amyotrophic lateral sclerosis (ALS) is categorized. For that reason, muscle twitching is usually interpreted as an early sign of ALS by the patients and their families, often increasing their demand for an early diagnosis.

2.1 Definitions and Causes

2.2. Clinical Presentation

In the case of hypothermia, relaxation, or extreme weakness of skeletal muscles of most, if not all impacted muscle groups, the disease of fasciculations will worsen. In view of a similar approach to hypersensitive actions occurring in ordinary hyper-reflexia, fasciculation frequency can be enhanced by excited physical and emotional situations such as tension, anxiety, exhaustion, and during rest. A significant difference exists between fasciculations and myokymia. Myokymia is an abnormal, spontaneous wave action under the skin, palpable by the examiner. Typically, they are less common and can be found in most any part of the organism. Peripheral nerve and muscle activities in ALS patients can also be uncovered by electromyography. Finally, fasciculations can be detected by physical investigation in almost all ALS patients, where the participants studied the inordinate sculpture of limb, oral, or thoracic muscles in the ALS clinic. To measure ailments, people are constantly complaining of "muscle fluttering." It looks like in ALS people to fasciculate. Others with MND announce a 65 to 90 percent, but slowed prevalence.

ALS muscle twitching or fasciculations are a clinical symptom that all practitioners will observe in their former patients with amyotrophic lateral sclerosis (ALS). Fasciculations are spontaneous, fine, and involuntary movements of muscles that occur in one or both eyelids, arms, fingers, feet, legs, and most prominently in the tongue, limbs, and abdominal muscles. In certain instances, they are noticed in the back or against the shoulders. Usually, fasciculations present singly, but multiple fasciculations can be seen in a particular session. The frequency and speed seem to be greater in body areas organized for finer action. Fasciculations are not noticed in slim, small muscle groups. On long and localized examination, it will become clear that only one upper skeletal muscle fasciculation has a single side.

3. Diagnostic Approaches

To recognize muscle twitching, many neurologists often use the paralyzed veteran rating scale as a clinical measure to record the presence of twitching as well as its localization along the entire course of the disease, while cleaning the patient's personal history. The awareness of muscle twitching should guide a correct approach in places with significant expertise in evaluation and early treatment of neuromuscular disorders. A repeated clinical observation may eventually prompt the need for more invasive investigation to argue a diagnosis of ALS. In proceeding in this direction, it is important to document the presence of tremors, excluding both the classic location of the benign subtype, as well as the presence of resting variant. To take into account in unavoidable cases of doubt opened by overt hand tremors are the significant proportion of patients presenting with isolated nuclear tremors while pronating arms and stretching fingers otherwise at rest. Their presence does not affect the TS disease size. For the sake of reaching a more accurate diagnosis, we should also mention that the rope tremor involving the left hand of a heavy smoker might originate electrodiagnostic studies appearing misleading in ruling out the presence of ALS. A detailed examination of the hand revealing excessive sweating should accompany such a clinical context.

Despite the relatively non-specific nature of muscle twitching, ALS muscle twitching should be accurately sought and recognized. The correct diagnosis of muscle twitching raises the possibility of an early invasive strategy to slow down the dissemination of the pathology, to eventually anticipate the initiation of neuroprotection. Moreover, muscle twitching is also recognized as a future research direction to disentangle the pathogenesis of disease origin and evolution.

3.1. Physical Examination

The threshold number of fasciculation potentials in a muscle divided by the duration of observation in minutes can help differentiate the etiology of fasciculation (e.g., ALS and myokymia) to some extent. While not universally accepted at all times, whether or not there are any validated scientific papers comparing results, this observation seems very relevant. The need to look for these signs does not even need to be stressed. They yield much information on the degree of involvement of the motor neuron, a prognostic element (in the absence of withdrawal times), and are, besides, an important warning signal. This has to be done in muscles that are severely involved and then repeated closer to the first date mentioned. The degree of these signs may define some requirements at follow-up in the management of ALS disease, but they play no defining role in the diagnosis of ALS.

The diagnosis of fasciculation or muscle twitching caused by amyotrophic lateral sclerosis (ALS) relies on the patient being evaluated at a healthcare facility, hospital, or with a specialist physician. It involves a careful physical examination, to some extent performed deliberately to elicit the characteristics typical of the disease fasciculation. As with any other medical condition, eliciting how the problem began plays a role in defining the cause. In the case of ALS, there is no such thing as an ALS mark on the body; thus, it is necessary to rely on a thorough physical examination as well as auxiliary tests, if needed. Several muscle twitching characteristics fasciculation were proposed by de Carvalho and Swash based on vast experience.

3.2. Electrodiagnostic Studies

In amyotrophic lateral sclerosis (ALS), the role of EDX is determinant. In a patient with clinically relevant upper motor neuron (UMN) and lower motor neuron (LMN) involvement (aka the ES-list), they have either upper and/or lower motor deficits and no better or combined alternative for explaining their weakness and atrophy. They have evidence from EMG studies of: A) neurogenic changes in the atrophic/distaved muscles with normal-appearing innervation muscles OR recruitment of low-threshold and large motor units in the least affected muscles; and B) marked numbers of fasciculation potentials or any fasciculation potentials in multiple muscles innervated by nerves that are clinically affected, muscle wasting with any clinical re-innervation.

In muscle twitching (fasciculations, F), EDX has the advantages of allowing concurrent movement recording, comparing motor units in the same muscle, and facilitating the diagnosis of myokymia, double discharges, neuromyotonia, and fasciculation potentials. On the downside, voluntary activation/normalization is necessary, and in 10% of fasciculations, the neurogenic feature is impossible to demonstrate.

Electrodiagnostic studies (EDX) are a specialized method for diagnosing peripheral nerve and muscle diseases. They target the function of the nerves (electroneurography, ENG, NCV) and muscles (electromyography, EMG), greatly complementing clinical history and neurological examination results. This three-dimensional view - combining information from history and bedside/examination findings with laboratory data - is essential for solving clinical problems.

4. Management Strategies

Rehabilitative Interventions: No studies to date have examined the effectiveness of physical aids or adaptations to reduce muscle twitching in people with ALS. Individuals with ALS often experience muscle twitching, which may be very annoying.

1. Management of Muscle Twitching in ALS Pharmacological Interventions: A number of drugs are available that may theoretically help to reduce or manage muscle twitching in ALS. Antispasticity drugs, including baclofen, tizanidine, and dantrolene, are designed to reduce the overactivity of the muscle, perhaps leading to less twitching; however, there is little evidence available regarding the effectiveness of these treatments in reducing muscle twitching. The use of drugs such as trihexyphenidyl (Artane) is sometimes used to reduce the severity or occurrence of muscle twitching but is not without significant side effects (e.g., cognitive impairment, precipitation of glaucoma, cardiovascular problems). Riluzole is the only licensed drug specifically for ALS, and it has been demonstrated to help maintain life over a longer period of time, following the onset of ALS; however, examination of specific studies indicated that it did not have significant benefit in the short term in relation to muscle twitching.

There is no cure for ALS, and as a consequence, the management of ALS sufferers is often a holistic and multifaceted approach in which pharmacological, rehabilitative, and assistive interventions are employed. These strategies are employed in an attempt to manage the muscle twitching, muscle weakness, loss of speech, swallowing, and breathing function that results from nerve cell (i.e., motor neurone) loss throughout the disease. Where muscle twitching is problematic for individuals, there are, however, a number of strategies that may be employed in an attempt to manage the symptom.

4.1. Medications

The use of effective antispastic agents should be done with care, avoiding overdosage, which may lead to decreased muscle strength and risk of pneumonia. Other medications may sometimes help, such as topical agents (lidocaine or capsaicin), tizanidine, valproate, gabapentin, topiramate, lamotrigine, dextromethorphan, mexiletine, and intramuscular botulism toxin. Clonazepam is quite effective in relieving fasciculations, especially at night, but it should be used with caution because of its possible depressant effects on respiration. Although good evidence for therapy may be lacking, people with ALS often seek information about potential relief and therefore an informed, individualized discussion with the physician is appropriate.

Pharmacotherapy may sometimes be helpful in relieving ALS muscle fasciculations, cramps, myokymia, stiffness, and spasticity. Although the FDA approved riluzole, edaravone, and recently cenobamate (XBIR-025) for treatment of amyotrophic lateral sclerosis, these were not approved for the control of cramps and fasciculations. These are the most common complaints of ALS patients. These muscle symptoms are among the most bothersome in ALS patients, but many studies have not well assessed the value of medications in the relief of these symptoms.

4.2. Physical Therapy and Exercise

Physical activity did not fulfill the needs of the body in terms of strength or improved resistance, and aerobic and stretching exercises had little to no effect on muscle power or improved resistance. Patients have been observed after exercising a feeling of increased well-being and redefining of physical function lost by various forms of decline. Exercise can also help to break down a coding dimension of the disease as a completely useless resistance, where all effort is doomed to fail. The positive feeling of participating in the treatment is able to alleviate personal and familiar depression, removing at least parts of the isolation of the patient from everyday life. In this way, the pain for the loss of some function affecting patients' attention might be shifted if not washed away by the hope for a future small and difficult recovery.

Physical therapy (PT) may improve functionality and maintain mobility during the ALS course, possibly modified by the site of onset. Resistance exercises may improve muscle strength, function, and survival despite the durability of such effects being uncertain. A personalized exercise regimen, considering the characteristics and evolution of clinical conditions and dystrophic problems, has the aims of maintaining functionality, providing a better quality of life, reducing weight loss, and reducing energy management problems. Physical therapy includes deep diaphragmatic (abdominal) breathing exercises, adequate techniques to fibrotic cough, and passive range-of-motion exercises. PT and respiratory exercise programs may improve the health-related quality of life in ALS patients. Nutritional support is able to improve respiratory and physical functions and may play an important role in nutritional status and resting energy expenditure in ALS patients, especially for those with increased resting energy expenditure.

5. Emerging Therapies

Two fascinating experimental classes describe emerging ALS treatments: SOD1 gene suppression, which has shown promise in phase I and II studies, and primate and now human studies of the BMAA and methyl-BMAA toxin counteractive diets. SOD1 mutations, known for causing a more severe and earlier-onset form of ALS, are found in 20% of fALS and in a small percentage of sALS cases (e.g. less than 2.5%). In phase I and II studies where SOD1 gene silencing was delivered with spinal route antisense oligonucleotides (ASOs) and adeno-associated viral vectors, the drug was shown to be well tolerated and effective at reducing spinal SOD1 protein runoff. Importantly, ALS participants and investigators in this first-in-human SNP trial do not know whether or not they have the SOD1 mutation. After ASOs, a simultaneous injection of spinal stem cells has batteries in vivo gene silencing shown to be safe. No significant side effects were found in short interviews with participants in the trial. The BMAA toxin has been one of many cyrexins reported in Guam in connection with the high prevalence of Seyin of all the various forms of ALS, but some link this to the diet of local people and the primate diet of the troop. In 178 ALS patients from the National Neurological Institute of Milan, Italy, BMAA levels were significantly higher in people with bulbar-onset and their cerebrospinal fluid. This study found a minor association between bulbar dysfunction (speech, swallowing, tongue, and arm and tongue injury), adjusted for motor features, ALSFRS-R average drawing.

Determination of the precision and duration of actions will be the next major steps for this drug.

Despite these disappointments, effective ALS disputing agents or experimental trials might exist within emerging applications. Lacosamide, a sodium channel blocker with the potential to reduce excitability, had received approval for ALS muscle cramping, based alone in small studies and preliminary case series. In a placebo-controlled, crossover study of just 40 patients, an R-Baclofen enantiomer known as arbaclofen or STX209 substantially decreased muscle twitching. A clinical trial of mavoglurant (AFQ056), a selective antagonist of the glutamatergic mGluR5 receptor, which reduced fasciculations in mouse studies, is predicted to be completed by March 2021. Vanillin, a byproduct found to knockdown SOD1 expression and reduce motor neuron loss in mice, had neuroprotective effects in a phase II study of large populations.

6. Quality of Life and Palliative Care

Muscle twitching can have an impact on quality of life via concern about progression of condition, making the patient's emotional well-being (feeling anxious, worried) a focal point of nascent research directions. This may resonate with the role of palliative care, whereby issues are 'managed' rather than 'cured', and 'family'/'environmental' care is recognized as an essential component of clinical care. An initial logic would, however, concede that respiratory difficulties, choking and shortage of breath, progressive muscle weakness, and potential dependency on ventilation would be first priorities for clinical intervention in order to adequately address a deteriorating quality of life. The recommendation and alternatives proposed on this basis, therefore, introduce our final comment on an important question that is known only too well: given that many chronic conditions have identified treatments and that rapidly targeting symptoms have become a focus of care, how does a condition continue to be labeled untreatable?

In lieu of a stand-alone management recommendation, we also consider the holistic aspects of managing this symptom by trying to answer whether muscle twitching can impact quality of life and also whether muscle twitching itself is a direct target for clinical intervention. In the first instance, the message is largely to reassure that muscle twitching in itself is not a common complaint but can be in the minority of individuals. In the second instance, the advice is also tempered by the fact that it is very unlikely to be a person's main problem and therefore questionable whether it would be worth focusing clinical efforts on this if there are other things under control and other symptoms to target. Instead, it might be more value-laden to start with a discussion as to how concerned a person is about muscle twitching and offering general advice on managing or ignoring it, which are likely the answers most people requiring a clinical service would expect.

7. Conclusion

In conclusion, understanding muscle twitching in ALS is a multi-dimensional task of great interest. The crucial role played by chronic and continuous denervation and reinnervation likely determines their characteristics and could also mask other, disease-nonspecific features they possess. Owing to the growing availability of open-access platforms that gather clinical, electrophysiological, and neuroimaging data, future work could also be based on data sharing and be performed in trait humans. The study of early treated ALS person may produce the first evidence supporting personalized, early symptomatic interventions for the disease.

This essay summarizes various aspects of ALS muscle twitching. These pathognomonic symptoms indicate the presence of motor neuron degeneration and are beginning to be used as efficacy measures in clinical trials. Although untoward, their frequency attenuates as the disease progresses. With one exception, all drugs used to treat other symptoms of ALS that were tested for their effect on muscle twitching showed no beneficial effect on them. Special interest is now attached to the potential use of registries to carry out large multi-center studies in trait instead of state humans. This type of research is expected to shed new light on information regarding the natural progression of ALS muscle twitching and the factors that influence it.

Understanding Muscle Twitching in ALS: Causes, Sensations, and Management

1. Introduction to ALS and Muscle Twitching

Amyotrophic lateral sclerosis (ALS), often referred to as "Lou Gehrig's disease," is a neurodegenerative condition that makes it difficult for neurons in your brain to communicate with motor units, which are the neurons that allow your muscles to contract (e.g. fibers). The ones that control all voluntary movement in your body. Among its first symptoms are twitching or spasm sensations that patients may experience. Practically everyone has experienced muscle twitch 'overnight' that seem to come from nowhere. Some well-defined 'hot spots' exist in several muscles, which are pretty common. It's that precise place you rub that seems too frequently to induce or forestall that jerk.

Now imagine if those twitches appear uninterrupted and in a lot more muscles. They may be regular or constant, with quick twitches of a muscle fiber visible. The sensation is often perceived by patients in two very different ways. Sensory nerves supply muscle all the time assessing the stretching or its length in order to give information to the brain on its positioning. By definition, they send information to the CNS when they feel a muscle is contracting (i.e. the muscle fiber is shortening). That's why they're often injured in sprain type accidents. The injury to those nerves averages out, and our awareness of muscle contractions goes on, but wane.

2. Understanding the Pathophysiology of Muscle Twitching in ALS

For understanding why muscle twitching occurs in ALS, it may be helpful to begin with the definition of the word twitch and then focus on the concept called 'fasciculation' as per its use in routine neuromuscular examinations. Twitch is a sudden movement caused by the contraction of a muscle or the muscles, commonly due to the activation of small motor units. A fasciculation is a similar small muscle contraction or muscle twitch, though it may be visible under the skin and this is often seen during neurological examination of the body. Fasciculations arise from the spontaneous firing of an individual motor unit, which is caused by subclinical hyperexcitability or instability of the lower motor neurons.

In ALS, the conditions that result in the fasciculation are heterogeneous and complex, involving the pathophysiological mechanisms causing reduced excitability in the subpopulation of the lower motor neurons. This reduced excitability occurs due to the imbalance of the normally high concentration of I(h) ion channels at the axonal/somatic/dendritic junction. Abnormal spread of hyperexcitability, remodeling of K and Na channels are other involved contributors. Various other intracellular, compartmental, and intra-injury stress networks also contribute to this new disturbing cell biology of the lower motor neurons that indicates that the abnormal fasciculations in ALS are a readout of a quite distressing internal microenvironment. On the other hand, the chronic female motor neurons in the bulbar trophic environment overexpress BDNF. This microenvironment has been demonstrated to generate equally distressful toxic motor neurons. The persistent IGF-1 cytonuclear dysbalance in motor neurons further adds to the negative environment responsiveness of specific neuromuscular junction in ALS. Since the ubiquitinated BDNF-60 pathway is particularly sensitive to neurogenesis in the function of anserine glutathione and plasma sulfur amino acids, malfunction and loss of GSH synthesis may play a critical role in promoting particular motor neuron vulnerability in female ALS cases and perhaps also in the protection of the neuromuscular junction. Successful neuromodification may not only revert the biophysical phenotype of lower motor neurons in their microenvironment, this could possibly also provide significant health benefits to respiratory onset lower motor neurons in ALS.

3. Common Symptoms and Sensations of Muscle Twitching in ALS

The traditional use and definition of the word "twitching" is when a single or very few muscle fibers contract, causing a very small visible "twitch" even under the hypodermic of the skin or over a large muscle mass. In ALS, the sensation of muscle twitching is described by many in different terms.

Describing the sensation of muscle twitching is quite varied from patient to patient. Sensations which are reported as muscle twitching in ALS include: "jumpy muscle", "tigger", "having a muscle jump or jerking upon waking", "the sensation of a constant internal buzz", "having a cell phone constantly vibrating in your pocket that doesn't stop", "fizzy", "bubbled feeling", "thumping", "popping", "maddening", and "pulse-like".

This symptom is also the largest factor in why individuals seek medical attention or further testing after experiencing a sensation they label as muscle twitching or who have attempted to stop the jerking sensation themselves before consulting with a medical professional.

When a person who suspects they have ALS presents for their first neurology office visit, very often the patient will be under the impression that what they feel by way of sensations in their muscles is unique or rare. This is not true; muscle twitching is not just one of the major and at times earliest symptoms in ALS but commonly described in other individuals who have a wide variety of other neurological disorders.

However, the speed in which muscle twitching and the related symptoms and weaknesses become more diffuse is a clue as to the likelihood of an underlying ALS concern versus another treatable neurological disorder.

4. Diagnostic Approaches for Muscle Twitching in ALS

The basic diagnostic challenge is to identify, understand, and relate the extent of fasciculations (muscle twitching) reported by the patient to what the examining clinician observes during a bedside test. Both the patient and clinician need to be aware of the range of forms that fasciculations can appear in. Patients should report all muscle twitching they experience in any location and any temporal-spatial setting, and the clinician needs to try to find specific fasciculations. Unfortunately, many patients report their fasciculations with no expectation of eliciting anything useful due to the facial reactions of clinicians who do not appreciate the basic, simple issues of patient acceptance with confirmation. The clinical examination forms the response to the patient's question, "What are my symptoms and what are they due to?" The fasciculation clinical examination is just advanced physiological muscle twitching.

We suggest that during the first interview, any patients' fasciculation symptoms are reported at length to the clinic, and we suggest that examination of facial muscles is essential to always confirm that the patient does report some fasciculation. We consider that the first office visit solves many problems for most of the patients' fasciculation information needs if the clinical examination is performed correctly. If the patient potentially has disease progression, such as ALS, the first step for the clinician is to very carefully confirm that the patient does have some fasciculations and provide clear visible confirmation of reports about which they are already clear and aware. For those patients who might be disappointed with the results, counseling should address the reasons why clinicians failed to provide objective supportive confirmation, if this was the case, with some explanation, understanding, and support. The first interview ultimately, if not immediately, differentiates the benign form of fasciculations that can always be ignored from the fasciculations associated with progressive disease, which are, of course, the pathological disease form.

5. Management Strategies for Muscle Twitching in ALS

Since muscle twitching is typically greatest during periods of rest, implementing a daytime schedule that is both varied and interesting may help decrease the focus on twitching awareness. Some patients find gentle, regular massage of affected muscle groups can be temporarily relaxing and lessen the sensation of twitching. At night, some patients find that a thick blanket on legs and feet adds needed sensory modulation. In keeping with its value in managing other types of spasticity, positioning and comfortable support of limbs during sleep may also be helpful. Warm baths, soft music, gentle massage, and warm milk may also help some patients sleep better. Medical management of painful muscle symptoms can be challenging. The symptoms require a targeted approach that is guided by cause. Where nerves are directly treated with localized intervention, medications haven't been very effective. Although antiseizure and muscle relaxant medications are frequently used to treat muscle symptoms, their effectiveness in a slow progressive condition such as ALS is often inconsistent.

5.1. Antiseizure Medications In an attempt to provide relief from painful muscle symptoms, physicians have administered antiseizure medications to patients with ALS. These are drugs that selectively dampen nerve activity and that have been successfully used to treat painful muscle problems in other settings. Although many physicians prescribe gabapentin for fasciculations even though it is only modestly helpful, patients work with their neurologist to adjust medications to their individual needs.

5.2. Muscle Relaxant Medications Medications that inhibit muscle spasticity are often used to treat painful muscle symptoms in ALS. These muscle relaxant drugs have been successfully used to treat painful muscle problems in other settings. Side effects like drowsiness and weakness can be dose-limiting, and persons who live with ALS need to adapt the timing and amount of medication to their daily routines. In the view of many, baclofen and tizanidine are more helpful in quelling the sensation of tightness than fasciculations. The decision to utilize an antiseizure or muscle relaxant medication and choice of specific agent are always guided by regular discussions with a patient's ALS center physician. These experts are in the best position to prescribe medications at safe and therapeutic doses.

6. Pharmacological Interventions for Muscle Twitching in ALS

When ALS patients experience muscle twitching that is bothersome or painful, medications can be considered. Patients should have a discussion with their ALS providers about the usefulness of starting a medication, as well as the possible side effects, drug interactions, and other instructions for use.

Reassuringly, many of the medications commonly used to treat muscle twitching symptoms in ALS have multiple uses and may be medications that patients are already taking. Prevention of painful, repetitive muscle contractions at the site of twitches or progressive disabling muscle spasticity is likely best accomplished with systemic, more constant levels of anti-spasticity agents. One aspect of medication response is now predictable—many, if not most, individuals taking muscle relaxant, weakly paralytic agents, such as benzodiazepines, experience a paradoxical activating adverse effect, which could be as disturbing as the twitch is and should be expected as a possibility, versus its seen benefit.

Consequences of twitching and spasticity present unique and compelling needs for the use of medication in PALS. They are emergent, without warning, and at all hours. Responses are needed immediately, always immediately, and sometimes at night. Over-the-counter agents and weak agents are insufficient to halt contractions quickly or effectively; thus, a strong agent must be discussed and prescribed to have quickly for emergencies. This pharmacological approach is now an option available for the partial management of both the clinical experience of involuntary muscle contractions; this knowledge of available types of therapeutic agents for each patient is a clinical potential for symptoms.

7. Non-Pharmacological Approaches for Managing Muscle Twitching in ALS

Triggers that are associated with an increased likelihood of muscle twitching include caffeine, being unwell (i.e., infection, especially fever), poor or change in sleep, pain, anxiety, stress, and dehydration. Keeping to a regular meal and fluid routine, regular affectionate contact with those who are important to you, and adequate exercise to your tolerance are also important to minimize your muscle twitching. Stress or anxiety management strategies such as breathing exercises, massage, or relaxation may also be helpful. Getting enough sleep is also an important factor in minimizing muscle twitching. For those who are having problems getting enough sleep, using relaxation techniques, using a transcutaneous (across the skin) electrical nerve stimulator (TENS) machine, or having a glass of milk are non-pharmacological options to consider.

Seeing a physiotherapist that has knowledge and experience with ALS and/or a neurologically educated myotherapist can be very beneficial, as they can assess and treat any muscle discomfort, and teach you how to stretch and move your muscles to best manage the discomfort and to minimize the likelihood of muscle twitching. Techniques such as acupressure and acupuncture performed by appropriately trained people, meditation, hypnosis, or other mind-body therapies may also be helpful in some people. Homeopathic or herbal therapies are also options that could be discussed with your doctor or ALS physiotherapist. Undergoing massage or reflexology may help to minimize muscle twitches for some people for a short period of time. A physiotherapist could teach your family member your muscle treatment regimen. Some people find warm water (e.g., swimming or a hot tub) or massage helpful in easing the sensation of muscle twitching, possibly because these activities provide sensory input to the nervous system, but the twitching can occur once out of the water or after massage has ceased. If you use a hot tub, be cautious of overheating as this can aggravate muscles for some people with ALS.

8. Physical Therapy and Exercise Recommendations for Muscle Twitching in ALS

People with ALS, and particularly those with muscle twitching and cramping, are sometimes reticent to exercise. They are not sure what may be too much or cause discomfort. However, exercise should be maintained in the face of muscle twitching as much as possible. It should be difficult (in fact, good) to push the body into a slight amount of fatigue without going too far. Exercise frequently and regularly will not escalate the twitching—what it may do is allow the muscle to experience a contraction that it is depending on twitching to do.

Physical Therapy

Physical therapy is often prescribed for those with muscle twitching, cramping, and ALS. The therapist may be able to identify certain movements that help relieve the shaky sensations or even assist in movement of the shaky muscle (such as tapping on the quad muscle to assist in extending the leg, which would relieve the shaky sensation of something pulling on the lower back). Use of cold and heat for muscle sensations can also be very beneficial and would be easily accessed using ice packs, heating pads, and warm water. Deep breathing, stretching, and slow constant movement throughout the day is beneficial.

9. Nutritional Considerations for Muscle Twitching in ALS

Nutritional management and appropriate levels of macro- and micronutrients play a key role in coping with muscle twitching in ALS. However, no specific recommendations exist because of the absence of scientific data. It is an area that remains unexplored, and future research should examine the effects of different nutrients on managing muscle twitching seen in ALS. It is highly recommended that ALS patients meet the general nutritional guidelines proposed by the Academy of Nutrition and

Dietetics, which are designed for individuals without ALS. These include consuming at least two cups of fruits and one cup of vegetables daily, eating a variety of whole-grain foods and minimizing consumption of highly processed grains, consuming a variety of protein foods, including seafood, lean meats, poultry, legumes (beans and peas), unsalted nuts, and seeds, and low-fat dairy options at each meal. It is advisable to limit food with added sugars such as sugar-sweetened beverages, limit sodium consumption, and select meals with reduced sodium. The focus should also be on consuming high-quality proteins and an adequate intake of healthy fats (olive oil, avocados, nuts, and seeds).

The action plan in coping with muscle twitching through a nutritional approach is to prioritize healthy eating, prioritize body weight preservation, and use modified textures when appropriate. It is advisable to consider certain symptoms and the structure and function of the chewing and swallowing mechanisms, as well as the potential effect of vitamin C in the mucus secretions. It is also important to select the appropriate food bulk, temperature, viscosity, and liquid content that can influence the difficulty of swallowing to keep them at a higher level. Depending on the stage of ALS and muscle weakness, it is also suggested to include a combination of texture-modified foods. High fiber content of fruits and vegetables should also be addressed when designing the diet of a patient with ALS, taking into account the prevalence of dysphagia in the study population. Increasing dietary fiber content is a common intervention to alleviate muscle twitching in ALS. The recommendations outlined in the Action Plan Section of The Role of Muscle Cramps in ALS: A Pilot Study are generally applicable to the limb, speaking, swallowing, facial, and jaw areas in patients with ALS. Therefore, dietitians are responsible for assessing and addressing muscle grain issues during a detailed assessment of patients' nutrition needs.

10. Emotional and Psychological Support for Individuals with Muscle Twitching in ALS

For individuals who are suffering from muscle twitching, the journey until they are diagnosed with ALS can be frustrating. The process is often long and may be filled with visits to different healthcare professionals, receiving a variety of tests, with many different possibilities being given. Patients can remain undiagnosed for several months, and in some cases, years. This can lead to frustration and impatience. To add stress to the situation, other people such as friends and family may not fully understand the symptoms that an individual is going through, often stating that they are "imagining" their muscle twitching. Friends and family may also begin to show concerns by asking questions that put pressure on the individual. Often the questions are left unanswered, which can have a negative impact on their mental health as well as the individual's. If you are in the diagnostic phase and undergoing tests but do not have a confirmed diagnosis, the strain may get to you as advice given may center around that specific diagnosis. For example, a doctor may say a person has a lumbar disc hernia or a gastrointestinal or neurological issue.

Individuals dealing with muscle twitching are often stressed due to multiple reasons:

- They are aware of the serious consequences associated with these muscle symptoms. The term "muscle fasciculation" or "twitching" often arises in the context of ALS. - They are frustrated due to a lack of good information and are waiting for results from doctor's visits. - They feel misunderstood, as others have difficulties understanding or are less interested to hear about the muscle twitching. - They notice that their mental status is not in line with how they "should" feel. - They experience physical voids: they are not sure which sport - if any - they can still participate in, they are worried about manual tests, but they are not sure if they should stop doing them. - They are confronted with long discussion groups full of "supplements" that allegedly could relieve the symptoms of fasciculation. - They feel alone in handling their complaints, and therefore they feel increasingly stressed by them.

So, please, keep the following advice in mind: We as human beings crave certainty, especially about our own health. We often begin the diagnostic process with symptoms yet without an understanding of where it will lead us.

11. Caregiver Tips and Support Strategies

Many patients with muscle twitching may experience anxiety, sleeplessness, and depression. Muscle twitching seems to be the most aggravating aspect for many ALS patients because it is so distressing to them. Although medications are usually not very helpful, counseling, physical therapy, and relaxation techniques are moderately effective at relieving the muscle twitching sensations. If stress and anxiety are contributing to muscle twitching, here are many emotional well-being perspectives to consider that may be helpful to patients. By learning what you can about muscle twitching, how to minimize them, and efficiently eliminating the ones that cause soreness, you play a vital role in your loved one's quality of life. Here are some helpful caregiving ways and action steps you can employ now to help your loved one and the care partner. If makes sure to remember your well-being along the way, all is more manageable in the long-haul.

There are various types of emotional support that can provide your loved one with a host of coping skills and examples of positive action. They are a patient to be able to do what they enjoy for as long as they want. Pre-located caregiver support groups can be an efficient source of help and there are other coaching and support groups provided without leaving home. Never hesitate to use all services to help minimize your workload, broaden your sense of responsibility, and support your emotional health. Home is the best place to be and it is important to make sure to know how to access citizen help. The importance of relying on your social and supportive network, including health professionals in the care team, will help make the patient's muscle twitching care more effective. The careful selection of vibrations could help assure an ample spectrum of social and emotional go-to support when you need it to be one of your vital long-term care strategies.

12. Research Advances and Future Directions in Muscle Twitching Management for ALS

Since ALS muscle twitching originates not in the motor endplates of NMJs but further back in the denervated muscle fibers, while the number of functioning motor units is in decline, the current ALS muscle twitching treatment is one of a functional management symptomatic approach. The focus of this article has been to explain what the sensations are of ALS muscle twitching, how to discriminate the muscle twitch from spasticity, and provide a relatively inclusive list of current modulating and management treatments in practical application. Relevant to this is the result from a meta-analysis paper that queried whether fasciculations had a prognostic value in defining ALS on presentation. It reported that fasciculations did indeed have a modest influence on predicting earlier diagnosis, as evidenced by RI and impedances at fifth intercostal breathing muscles and median motor conduction velocities across post elementary recruits reporting on the suspected time of symptom onset. Their report concluded that evidence exists for the premise that the presence of fasciculations can increase the level of diagnostic certainty.